LITTLE
PILATES

THE LITTLE BOOK OF PILATES

Copyright © Summersdale Publishers Ltd, 2023

An Hachette UK Company
www.hachette.co.uk

Vie Books, an imprint of Summersdale Publishers Ltd
Part of Octopus Publishing Group Limited
Carmelite House
50 Victoria Embankment
LONDON
EC4Y 0DZ
UK

www.summersdale.com

Printed and bound in the UK

ISBN: 978-1-80007-695-2

The
LITTLE BOOK OF
PILATES

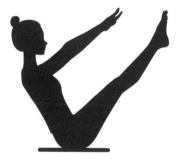

Rachel Lawrence

Contents

Introduction

Welcome to the world of Pilates. In this book you will learn everything you need to know about the Pilates method and how you can use it to get the best out of your mind and body. Created just over 100 years ago, Pilates is a unique system of exercises that will increase your strength and flexibility as well as your mind/body awareness to help you feel calmer, happier, more in control of your body and more comfortable in your own skin. Popular with dancers, athletes, royalty and celebrities the world over, Pilates is a great way to improve fitness through structured exercises that you learn and repeat, building your core strength, spinal flexibility and overall fitness as well as knowledge of your own body. It teaches you to be more mindful of your movement and to focus on the quality of each movement rather than the quantity. Less is more with Pilates!

No matter what your experience or fitness level, this book is for you. With clear instructions and guidance, you can take yourself on a journey that's tailored to you. From Beginners to Advanced, here you will find everything you need to practise Pilates confidently at home. Starting today you will be on your way to a fitter, healthier, happier you!

IN 10 SESSIONS YOU WILL
FEEL THE DIFFERENCE,
IN 20 YOU WILL SEE
THE DIFFERENCE, AND
IN 30 YOU'LL HAVE A
WHOLE NEW BODY.

Joseph Pilates

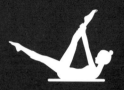

CHAPTER ONE:
THE PILATES SYSTEM

Pilates was originally called Contrology
because its creator Joseph Pilates was an
advocate of teaching the mind to master
the body. This method will help you gain
mastery over your muscles and breath – and
ultimately your fitness. In this chapter you
will learn the background to Pilates and
the key principles to begin your practice.

WHO WAS JOSEPH PILATES?

Joseph Hubertus Pilates was born in Germany in 1883; his father was a prize-winning gymnast of Greek descent and his mother a naturopath. Growing up in an environment of fitness and alternative medicine greatly influenced the young Joseph. He threw himself into exercise at an early age to overcome asthma, rickets and rheumatic fever. By the age of 14 he was modelling for anatomy magazines, such was his physical stature. With a keen interest in all types of movement he practised body building, gymnastics and diving, as well as studying Eastern and Western forms of exercise and philosophy.

By 1912, he had moved to the UK and was working as a fitness instructor, boxer and circus performer; he's also rumoured to have led self-defence training at UK Police Headquarters, Scotland Yard. When World War One broke out he was interred in a camp on the Isle of Man with other German nationals, and it was here he began to develop his own ideas for movement practices and metal spring-based apparatus to help rehabilitate the injured and disabled. In 1926 he travelled to New York by ship, meeting his wife Clara on board and together they set up the first Pilates Studio in New York City. This became a haven for a diverse mix of high society, film stars, elite athletes and performers, but it was the dance community who really embraced his movement system. Famous choreographers such as George Balanchine and Martha Graham would regularly send their dancers to him for rehabilitation from injury as well as to improve their athletic ability.

During his long career Joseph Pilates created over 600 exercises for the apparatus he invented, as well as 34 distinct matwork exercises, all of which are featured in this book and still form the basis of most twenty-first-century Pilates lessons. Joseph regarded his movement method as a path to good health through mental well-being as well as physical fitness. And it is this holistic approach to exercise, in particular – the way his method can be adapted to suit anyone – which has made it so appealing today.

JOSEPH PILATES' LEGACY

Joseph Pilates' work was carried on by a small group of practitioners known as the "Pilates Elders". This group of men and women were trained directly by Joseph and Clara Pilates, and they went on to set up their own studios leading to different schools of training and different styles of the original movements. From the Elders, hundreds and now thousands of Pilates instructors have been trained all over the world. In more recent years, the method has been recognized for its rehabilitative benefits by the sports science community. This has led to a wealth of instructors offering their expertise from a huge diversity of backgrounds from dance to physiotherapy, each contributing their own "take" on the movements much as the Elders did. With more scientific knowledge the original exercises have been adapted and improved over time to allow for increased understanding of human anatomy and how it functions. But the fundamentals of Joseph Pilates' exercises remain the same.

In the original Pilates studio Joseph taught both his matwork programme and a more comprehensive programme on the specialized apparatus he invented. With wondrous names such as the Reformer, Cadillac, Wunda Chair and Ladder Barrel, they are still very much part of a fully equipped studio today.

Pilates has become synonymous with well-being, good health and a balanced lifestyle. With the explosion of social media, Pilates has moved firmly into the mainstream with film stars, celebrities and sports stars regularly posting pictures of themselves mid-workout and glowing with health.

Joseph Pilates' dream was to see his method reach out beyond the elite to the general population so that everyone could benefit from it. The fact you are reading this book today is testament to how much he has influenced the fitness and well-being industry. With that in mind, allow this book to take you on a journey through the principles, the exercises and holistic intention behind the method; everything you need for a happier, healthier life.

THE SIX KEY PRINCIPLES OF PILATES

Joseph Pilates was deeply committed to his exercise method and through his legacy, key components of how he taught have become guiding principles for all schools of teaching. These are the six principles of his method.

1. Breath

Useful as a stress reliever as well as an aid to the exercise itself, the breathwork in Pilates is a vital component of every movement. Master the breathing and you'll master the exercise! It helps you focus, relax into the movement pattern and most importantly activate the deep core muscles (see page 34) that are such a key part of the Pilates technique.

Pilates uses the lateral breathing method (see page 38) to emphasize the expansion sideways of the rib cage, utilizing the intercostal (rib) muscles while maintaining a consistent yet gentle inward pull of the abdominals. The benefits of this are more oxygen in the body, decreased stress, lower blood pressure, core activation and better circulation. Lateral breathing is the opposite of natural breathing and can take a while to get the hang of, but it is worth it. In fact, the breathing alone is great exercise for increasing core strength and it's a good idea to spend some time learning it before you begin the exercise programme.

Pilates uses both set breath patterns and active breathing. Set breath patterns are where you will coordinate your breath with a particular part of the movement; this not only enhances your focus as well as relaxation, but it is to encourage you not to hold your breath. Holding your breath can create tension in the muscles and Pilates is all about releasing tension while building strength and flexibility. Active breathing can radically change the dynamic of an exercise. It is a rhythmic form of breathing which can take on different speeds and force, and will change the feel and intensity of the movement. It can be quite percussive for some exercises and gentle for others, and is something to master for the ultimate sense of well-being and control over your body.

2. Concentration

An awareness of what you're doing in the moment, and what you're doing next allows you to focus on the movement and increase the mind/body connection. This is also a great stress reliever and one of the reasons Pilates is often called "mindful movement". You are literally tuning your mind and body into moving in harmony. The more you concentrate on the exercise, the more you will benefit from the movement. By thinking about the movement, what muscles you are using, what the breath pattern is and where you want to feel it you will quickly gain mastery over your body. It is these elements that will improve your health and fitness as well as lead to a calmer state of mind. The ideal is for you to perform the exercise to the best of your ability and as correctly as your knowledge and fitness level allow - you'll find all the tips and cues you need in the exercise section of this book.

Do try to spend some time each day focusing on being in the moment; it can be anywhere, anytime – while out for a walk or making a coffee. Just allow yourself to completely focus on the "now", the task at hand, and eliminate all the other chatter in your head. How do you feel? How are you moving? How does it feel to move? This is a great way to start building an awareness of your body. Try to build up your concentration levels, because it's important to maintain focus continually throughout a Pilates session. While practising Pilates it's important to continually go inward, assess how you're doing, correct your alignment, and at all times be kind and patient with yourself. That way you will reap the benefits of the practice.

3. Centre

Centre refers to several concepts in Pilates; your centre of gravity, your core which is at the centre of your body and a sense of being centred in your movement. Throughout all the Pilates exercises you will need to find your centre of gravity; that point where you feel in balance, in control and stable. Gravity varies from person to person because everyone is built differently with each body being unique. While some people may find certain exercises easy, others will not. This is not a failing, far from it, it is often simply that they may need to shift their centre of gravity by adjusting their position in a movement to make the exercise more achievable. Keeping centred throughout your movement by having adequate stabilization is all down to body awareness and most importantly core strength.

The core muscles are without doubt at the heart of all Pilates movements – consisting of the abdominals, back muscles, gluteal muscles and pelvic floor.

Strengthening them, maintaining that strength and learning to control it is what sets Pilates apart from other exercise methods. You work from the core out to the limbs. Each exercise begins with a set up, then the breath, followed by core activation and finally the movement. It sounds very complicated but you will soon find it second nature. Think of it when you are watching world class athletes start a race: they arrive at the starting line, they get themselves into position, adjusting their bodies as needed so they feel in the best place to begin. They take a breath, they mentally focus and wait for the starting signal and then they are off, perfectly prepared for what is to follow. It's a ritual and this is how to think of your own Pilates practice: take your time, find your centre, connect to your core and what follows will be a wonderfully beneficial practice.

4. Control

The ability to control your body through a movement with a sense of confident relaxation rather than tension is essential to Pilates. When attempting new forms of exercise or unknown movements it is very common to tense up, to over-recruit the muscles or to simply try too hard, all of which leads to excessive tension in the body. In Pilates we look for relaxed control; learning to perform the movements with both effort and ease. This may sound contradictory but it is achievable and the way to reach this level of skill is through regular and consistent practise.

It takes time to build control of the body and it takes patience. Like any skill, you learn Pilates through practise, through making mistakes and trying again, and you repeat, repeat, repeat. Each time you repeat a movement, you are improving your strength, your flexibility and building a greater sense of control over your body.

Control is very much a skill you can only learn by "doing". If you look at any skilled mover such as a dancer or gymnast there is a sense of ease, control and grace in what they do and that is because they have reached – through years of practice – a level of expertise in the control of their body. This is what you are aiming for. Pilates will feel awkward at first, just as it would for anyone learning a new skill, but with practice and repetition you will soon grow your skill and confidence. The benefits of this are huge, not only will it advance your practice but you will notice how much easier everything physical in your life becomes. So, practise, practise, practise!

5. Precision

Precision means paying attention to the exact details of each exercise and the breath pattern, and it's what sets Pilates apart from other exercise systems. There are many exercises in Pilates that will look similar to exercises you have seen before, but it is the way that you do them that makes the difference. A Pilates approach is a precise one: it is about having an understanding of the way your body is moving, staying as close to the instructions for movement and breathing as possible, and most importantly having the patience to learn and improve your practice. Fundamentally, Pilates is about understanding the exercise on a deeper level which is why it is often referred to as intelligent movement. You can be assured that the more precise you are and the deeper your understanding, the stronger, more skilful and more flexible you will become.

Our bodies are all different: we move in different ways and over time we build up unhealthy postural habits; the way we stand, sit at our computer, or indeed play sport.

Many sportspeople are what we call one-sided, meaning they have great strength and control on one side of their body, the dominant side – think of a tennis player or football striker – but are less strong on the other side of their body. Professional athletes have help with this, in fact many do Pilates for that very reason. While it's less pronounced outside of elite sportspeople, we all have a dominant side and a less developed side. The precision used in Pilates seeks to rebalance the body; undo incorrect movement patterns, build equal strength and flexibility and re-educate your muscles on moving your body in a more efficient and safe way. The controlled and precise movements of Pilates enable the neural pathways to reset, the motor control to improve and the mind-body connection to strengthen. From this precision everything can flow.

6. Flow

In Pilates, flow means the activation of muscles at just the right timing to create a fluidity of movement. Strength comes in many forms and one of those is the ease with which you move. To create flowing, graceful movement requires all the previous principles integrating together for one seamless workout. It's often the case that people see a Pilates move, think it's easy and then try it only to find themselves stopping and starting, losing their balance or just unable to move in the same way. This is where flow comes in. Once you understand the exercises, you are looking to create a sense of flow within each movement and ultimately a flow from one movement to the next, so your Pilates workout becomes one long flowing session. This brings everything together: a calm mind, a calm body, a body perfectly at ease with movement and a balanced workout routine that will leave you feeling refreshed, strong, flexible and ready for life.

All six of the key principles of Pilates need to be present when executing the exercises in this book, no matter what your level or ability. What links them all is the element of both mind and body integrating together.

As an individual you can choose how you want to integrate these principles. You may choose to emphasize more of the physical aspect to improve muscle tone, core strength or rehabilitate from injury. Alternatively, you may choose to focus on the mindful element to relieve stress, anxiety and unwanted tension. Ultimately you will move through a process of focused learning and execution of movement that will benefit you for the rest of your life. Now you have read the key principles let's get you prepared for your practice.

JUST TRY NEW THINGS. DON'T BE AFRAID. STEP OUT OF YOUR COMFORT ZONES AND SOAR.

Michelle Obama

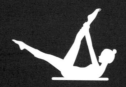

CHAPTER TWO: GETTING STARTED IN PILATES

This chapter will tell you everything you need to know in order to prepare for your practice. How you practise, where and for how long is all your choice but, ultimately, this is about creating the right setting for you to get the absolute best out of your time on the mat.

SETTING UP YOUR HOME STUDIO

Find a place in your home which is a calm, comfortable, space you can relax in. It can be a room or simply a place dedicated to your practice, which has no distractions and where you can be alone and uninterrupted. In creating a fun ritual of a place to go, you will quickly find yourself looking forward to your time on the mat. This will help train your mind and body that when you are in this space you can switch off from everything else to focus on yourself. If you can, place a large mirror in the space so you can see yourself – this will help you to correct your alignment during the session. Be sure the space is big enough to extend your arms and legs in all directions without hitting the furniture; you don't want to keep shuffling around to make space to do the movements! The most essential item in this space will be your Pilates mat.

BUYING YOUR FIRST PILATES MAT

Pilates really focuses on the movement of the spine in all directions, therefore it is essential to invest in a good quality Pilates mat to support and cushion the spine during your practice. Pilates mats are thicker than yoga mats which is why it is not recommended to use a yoga mat. For Pilates you want to purchase a mat that is 8–15mm thick. They tend to be more expensive than yoga mats because of this, but a good quality mat will last you a long time, and most importantly take care of your body. You can buy mats which roll up or fold up, ideally you want to buy one that is made of sustainable material, non-slip and long enough that you can lie down fully without having to shuffle around. Having a good quality mat will elevate your practice as well as protect your spine.

WHAT TO WEAR

In Pilates, much attention is paid to the alignment of your spine and joints so it is ideal if you can wear clothing that is comfortable and close fitting, in order to check your position in the mirror. Being able to see the body and getting to understand movements in such a way that you can analyse yourself anatomically will be of immense benefit, and help reduce any anxiety about how you look. Invest in an outfit that makes you feel great, is made from fabrics which allow the skin to breathe and that you feel completely at ease in. Most practitioners wear leggings and close-fitting sports tops, or shorts and t-shirts. You will get hot during your practice so be sure to wear something cool and practise in bare feet to encourage connection to the floor and a feeling of being grounded throughout your practice.

CONSULT YOUR DOCTOR

Pilates is a wonderful exercise regime suitable for everybody, but it is vital if you have any medical issues to check with your doctor before starting. There are certain medical conditions that aren't compatible with some of the traditional Pilates exercises so it is important to consult a medical professional if you have any doubts whatsoever. Two key conditions are pregnancy and osteoporosis.

Pregnant women can do a modified Pilates programme to support their body as they transition through pregnancy, however these are specialized programmes which are not covered in this book. Please do not attempt these exercises if you are pregnant.

If you have osteoporosis, do check in with your doctor before starting a Pilates programme. You must avoid all exercises with spinal flexion - rounding forward of the spine, forward bending and rotation. These can put you at risk of compression fractures. Instead, focus on extension exercises, core work on your side, kneeling exercises and exercises lying on your front.

UNDERSTANDING YOUR SPINE – A QUICK ANATOMY LESSON

Did you know your spine can move in seven different directions? Forward, back, side bend right, side bend left, rotating right, rotating left and finally, axial elongation where the spine lengthens vertically to improve posture for greater mobility, stability and good health. In Pilates this is always the focus of your practice so let's do a brief overview to get you better acquainted.

The spine is made up of 33 bones called vertebrae. They are stacked one on top of the other to form a column with natural curves that help absorb the shock of movement. They range in size and have five sections, three of which are responsible for the primary movement of the spine. From the top they are the Cervical spine, consisting of seven vertebrae beginning from below the head to the base of the neck. These are the smallest bones and essential for moving the head and neck. Below this is the Thoracic spine consisting of the next 12 vertebrae, which increase in size as they go down, finishing at the bottom rib. They move individually with the ribs and are essential for movements of the upper back. The Lumbar spine are the next five vertebrae starting from below the bottom rib to the pelvis. These are the strongest and largest of the vertebrae, responsible for movements of the lower back and essential for their weight-bearing abilities. The Sacrum consists of five fused vertebrae (in adults) that form a triangular shape with each side connected to a hip bone. This has a huge influence on the alignment of the lower back and stability of the pelvis. And finally, the Coccyx which consists of three to five bones which articulate with the Sacrum and are a key point of attachment for many muscles and ligaments.

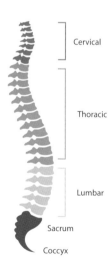

Cervical

Thoracic

Lumbar

Sacrum

Coccyx

WHERE AND WHAT IS THE CORE?

The core is a group of muscles between the base of your rib cage and your hip bones in the front, and down to the base of your buttocks at the back. Imagine it like a box containing everything you need to move. Whether to initiate action, or to stabilize the body while action takes place, these are the key muscles we focus on in Pilates. Here's a quick guide to their names and what they do.

Abdominals

Recognized for the aesthetic benefit of flattening and sculpting the waistline, the abdominals are a group of four muscles that create forward bending (flexion), rotation and side bending of the body. *Transversus abdominus* is the deepest muscle and one we focus on consistently in Pilates. When contracted it acts like a corset to stabilize, support and protect the spine and plays a vital role in posture. *Rectus abdominis* otherwise known as the six pack is the central section of your abdomen which contracts to create forward flexion of the spine. The external obliques are found on both sides of the body and are involved in forward flexion, as well as side bending and rotation to the opposite side. Internal obliques are deeper in the body, also on both sides, and create forward flexion, side bending and rotation to the same side.

Spinal Extensors

These are found on the back of the body and can be divided into three groups: the erector spinae, semispinalis and deep posterior spinal group. They serve to extend the spine when they contract. Strengthening them is vital for preventing back injuries, supporting osteoporosis and successful return to activity post back injury. They also assist in side bending and rotation.

Gluteus Maximus and Pelvic Floor Muscles

The gluteus maximus are the powerful buttock muscles used in activities such as running and walking but they also play a vital role in posture, helping to maintain core stability. And finally, the pelvic floor is a muscular sling that sits at the bottom of the abdominal cavity supporting the internal organs.

BEST PRACTICE

It is recommended you exercise on an empty stomach or leave at least two hours between eating and exercising. Pilates has a high amount of core work, which means you will be compressing your abdominals consistently for the time you are moving so be sure to leave time to digest your food! Staying hydrated is important too; drink plenty of water before, after and during class.

Remember that you are about to start a whole new way of moving your body and integrating your mind – with this there will inevitably be a transition process that takes place. You may find your mind and body reacting in unexpected ways: frustration, cramp in your legs, or you may not feel anything is happening at all, but Pilates is a slow burn method. Keep going, don't give up and the changes will come. Pilates is so much more than exercise, it's a whole way of being.

HOW TO USE THE EXERCISE SECTIONS IN THIS BOOK

For ease of use and understanding, the exercises in this book have been organized into three chapters: Beginners, Intermediate and Advanced. No matter what your level of fitness it is important you start at the beginning, in order to build your technique and practice. Once you can do all the beginner exercises competently, you can add intermediate exercises one by one, and so on to the advanced. Each exercise has been broken down into three sections to help you learn it thoroughly. The Movement section describes the set-up position, the move itself, breath pattern and suggested repetitions of the exercise. The Benefits section explains what you will gain from the exercise. The Tips and Technique Cues are there to help you achieve, modify, or increase the challenge to suit you. Before you start, be sure to learn the Pilates breathing technique, neutral placement of your spine, and always begin with a warm-up and end with a cool down!

LATERAL BREATHING

To get you started on connecting to your core it is recommended you spend time practising the Pilates breathing method. You will use this breathing technique throughout your practice and it is important to make sure you can feel the connection before you start the beginners' programme.

Stand in front of a mirror and place your hands on the sides of your ribs. Take a long deep inhale through your nose and at the same time try to expand your ribs sideways into each hand. Now take a long, steady exhale and allow your ribs to relax beneath your hands and move inwards toward each other. You want to practise this regularly and aim for being able to inhale for the count of five and exhale for the count of five. Relax your shoulders and neck, and try to visualize the motion of your ribs moving sideways on the inhale and coming together on the exhale.

Once you feel comfortable with this, you can add the next layer of movement. Still in front of the mirror, gently pull in the lower abdomen; an easy way to feel this is to pull your navel inwards and slightly upward toward your spine. This is a contraction of the abdominal muscles and what you will see in the mirror is the flattening out of this area. Now try to hold that contraction gently while you inhale, this will start to stabilize your pelvis and spine. As you exhale, draw those muscles in and deepen the contraction without allowing your pelvis to move. Now you will be feeling the *Transversus abdominus* muscle working to keep your spine and pelvis still. Keep practising until you feel in control, and, most importantly, do not worry. This is generally the most challenging aspect of Pilates for people new to the practice. It will take time to learn, time to tune into the mind/body connection. So go easy on yourself!

Warm-Up – Pelvic Curl

The Movement

1. Start position. Lie on your back with your knees bent and feet hip-width apart. Find your neutral position by aligning both your hip bones and pubic bone; visualize the area between these three points like the surface of a bucket of water with you trying to keep the liquid from spilling out. Place your arms by your side, palms down. This is the start position you'll use at the beginning of all exercises on your back.

2. Exhale. Start to pull your abdominals in and tip your imaginary bucket backward as if to spill the water over your chest. When you can't tip any further, curl your spine up off the mat, moving through lower, middle and upper back until you feel the weight on the back of your shoulders. This is the bridge position. If you can see yourself in a mirror, you are looking for a straight line from your knees to your ribs.

3. Inhale. Hold the position.

4. Exhale. Slowly lower your spine back onto the mat, moving sequentially through the spine, pelvis and finally tailbone returning to your neutral position.

5. Repeat the sequence 8–10 times.

The Benefits

Strengthens the core, legs, hips and glutes. Improves spinal mobility and articulation. Releases tension in the back.

Tips and Technique Cues

- Start to pull the abdominals in before moving the spine to encourage the core to work as separate from the movement.

- Keep your knees hip-width apart throughout as this will tone and strengthen your inner thigh muscles.

- Visualize peeling your spine up off the floor one vertebra at a time and then laying it back down in the same way.

- Keep the ribs down when the body is in the bridge position so as not to arch your back.

Warm-Up – Spine Twist Supine

The Movement

1. Start position. Lie on your back and raise your legs one at a time into the tabletop position: knees gently pressed together and held directly above the hips with lower legs parallel to the floor, feet gently pointed and arms out to the side with palms facing up.

2. Exhale. Gently pull your abdominals in and tilt your pelvis just a little toward your face so you feel your core muscles engage.

3. Inhale. Rotate your pelvis and legs as one unit to the right, keeping knees together and shoulders on the mat.

4. Exhale. Draw your abdominals in and rotate back to the start position.

5. Inhale. Rotate your lower body to the left.

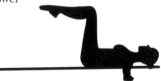

6. Exhale. Return once again to your start position.

7. Repeat 4–5 times in each direction making a total of 8–10 times.

The Benefits

Strengthens all the core muscles. Also strengthens the inner thigh muscles, the quads and the calf muscles. Improves spinal rotation of the body while teaching control of the lower back muscles which can help protect the spine from injury when using rotation in day-to-day activities or during dynamic sports activities.

Tips and Technique Cues

- Focus on pulling the abs in before rotating the torso.

- Keep squeezing the legs together gently so you move the whole lower body as one unit.

- Keep the knees aligned with the centre of your pelvis.

- Keep both shoulders on the mat.

- Try not to let the feet drop, use your thigh muscles to hold the legs in their 90-degree, right-angle position throughout the exercise.

Warm-Up – Chest Lift

The Movement

1. Start position. Lie on your back in the neutral position, knees bent, feet hip-width apart. Place hands behind head, elbows pointing out within your peripheral vision.

2. Exhale. Curl your head and chest up until your shoulder blades have lifted off the mat.

3. Inhale. Hold the position.

4. Exhale. Draw the abdominals in and return to the mat.

5. Repeat 5–10 times.

The Benefits

This movement teaches you how to effectively engage the deep core muscles.

Tips and Technique Cues

- Draw your abdominals in before lifting the head and chest to encourage activation of the Transversus Abdominus muscle.

Warm-Up –
Chest Lift with Rotation

The Movement

1. Start position. This exercise begins from the top position of the Chest Lift (step 2 on page 44).

2. Exhale. Rotate your head, chest and torso to one side. Inhale. Rotate back to centre.

3. Exhale. Rotate to the opposite side.

4. Inhale. Rotate back to centre. Continue this rotation alternating sides 6–10 times while keeping the head, chest and torso lifted. Exhale. Lower your head, chest and torso back down onto the mat.

The Benefits

Develops the oblique muscles which are vital for sculpting the waistline and helping to prevent lower back injury.

Tips and Technique Cues

- Keep your head, neck and chest lifted, maintaining the same height throughout the exercise.

Warm-Up – Leg Lift Side

The Movement

1. Start position. Lie on one side with your bottom arm extended straight above your head, with your head resting on it. Place your other arm, palm down in front of your chest, fingers parallel to your body. You are trying to find a side lying neutral position by having your hips stacked one above the other.

2. Exhale and raise both legs off the mat, keeping them together and maintaining a straight line through your body.

3. Inhale to lower the legs to the start position. Repeat 8-10 times then change to the other side and repeat.

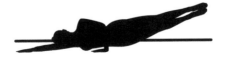

The Benefits

Strengthens the lower spinal flexors, abdominal obliques, tones inner and outer thigh muscles. Most importantly, teaches core stability for the lateral flexors of the spine.

Tips and Technique Cues

- Visualize you are lying between two panes of glass so you are completely on your side.

- Think of reaching the legs out as you lift and avoid rolling forward or back.

- Keep the legs pressing together throughout the movement.

- To increase the level of difficulty, try lowering the legs but not quite touching the mat in between repetitions.

- If you feel discomfort in your lower back bring your feet forward and focus on pulling the abdominals in throughout to reduce the tendency to overuse the back muscles.

Warm-Up – Back Extension

The Movement

1. Start position. Lie on your front with forehead on the mat, arms by your side, palms pressing onto your thighs. Legs together with feet gently pointed.

2. Exhale to lift the head, upper and middle back off the mat, keep the palms pressing into your legs and keep your legs together.

3. Inhale to slowly lower the body back to the start position.

4. Repeat 8–10 times.

The Benefits

Strengthens the spinal extensors while practising the ability to contract abdominals to support the lower back.

Tips and Technique Cues

- Maintain abdominal contraction through your exhale and gently press your pelvis forward into the mat to prevent overuse of lower back muscles.

- Keep the legs together and down on the mat throughout the movement.

- Visualize your spine lifting one vertebra at a time in a gentle, even curve.

- Try to create an even movement down through the neck and into the upper and mid back.

THE BEGINNING IS THE MOST IMPORTANT PART OF THE WORK.

Plato

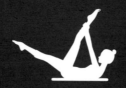

CHAPTER THREE: BEGINNERS' EXERCISES

This chapter will teach you ten fundamental exercises which are a great workout on their own, as well as a warm-up for a longer, more advanced programme. Take your time and think of it like learning a language: keep repeating until you fully understand. Now, roll out your mat and let's begin.

The Hundred

The Movement

1. Start position. Lie on your back, legs in tabletop position, arms by your side, palms down on the mat.

2. Exhale to draw your abdominals in and raise your head and chest up off the mat, eyeline forward. At the same time float the arms up so they are beside your body and parallel to the floor.

3. Inhale for the count of five while simultaneously pumping the arms down and up on each count.

4. Exhale for the count of five while simultaneously pumping the arms down and up on each count. Do this for 10 rounds of breathing.

5. Lower the upper and lower body back on to the mat.

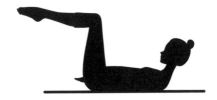

The Benefits

Increased core stability, abdominal strength. Improved breathing, breath control and endurance. Strengthens hip flexors, thigh, shoulder and arm muscles.

Tips and Technique Cues

- Keep eyeline forward and chin slightly nodded to reduce neck tension: if it is too much for your neck, put your head down and continue.

- Keep the elbows straight throughout and reach your fingertips forward.

- To increase the challenge further, straighten the legs: firstly straight up toward the ceiling then if you wish to advance even further lower them to a position you can hold without your back arching.

- If you feel your back arching lift your legs or bend the knees.

- To increase the challenge, add active breathing; inhaling five times and out five times in a percussive rhythm for 10 repetitions. This is why it is called the Hundred as it creates 100 breaths.

One Leg Circle

The Movement

1. Start position. Lie on your back with arms out to the side, palms up and legs straight. Bend your right knee and extend the leg, gently pointing your toes toward the ceiling. Flex the foot on your left leg.

2. As you exhale, "draw" a circle with your right leg, allowing your pelvis to lift off the mat as the leg moves left across the body, then letting your pelvis return to the mat as the leg circles right and back up to the start position.

3. Inhale to repeat the movement. Do this sequence five times then change direction, starting by going outward on the exhale. Repeat sequence five times. Then switch to the left leg and repeat from the beginning.

The Benefits

Hip mobility and release. Strengthens all the abdominal muscles as well as the spinal muscles that rotate and stabilize the body. Also works the hip, knee and ankle muscles.

Tips and Technique Cues

- Be sure to draw the abdominals in so there is neither excessive arching nor flattening of the back as the leg moves – focus on feeling the core stabilize the pelvis while allowing it to rotate gently with the leg movement.

- If you are unable to straighten your legs due to tight hamstrings, bend your knee as much as you need to.

- Keep the movement and breath as even as you can.

- Aim to pause momentarily between each circle.

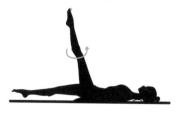

Roll Up

The Movement

1. Start position. Lie on your back on the mat, legs straight and gently pressing together, feet pointed. Arms straight and overhead, palms facing up.

2. Inhale as you move your arms forward followed by a lift of the head and chest.

3. Exhale to draw the abdominals in and lift further, curling your spine up off the mat and reaching toward your toes in a seated position.

4. Inhale to begin rolling back down until you feel your sacrum on that mat.

5. Exhale to finish the movement and bring your arms back overhead. Repeat 10 times.

The Benefits

Strengthens the abdominals and the hip flexors. Improves spinal mobility and flexibility of both hamstrings and lower back.

Tips and Technique Cues

- If you are unable to come up with your legs straight, modify by bending your knees and if needed place your hands underneath your knees for support to assist with the lift up.

- Keep the movement as smooth as possible, visualizing moving through each vertebra.

- Avoid excessive momentum with your arms and keep your shoulders relaxed throughout.

- Imagine trying to lift up and over a ball in your lap so you continue to draw the abdominals in throughout the movement.

- If you have the flexibility you can place your palms down on either side of your legs in the upright position. Avoid letting your head drop below your arms.

- An alternative if the stretch aspect is too challenging is to come up until your shoulders are directly above your hips, inhale and then return to the mat on the exhale. Repeat 8–10 times.

Spine Stretch

The Movement

1. Start position. Sit upright on your mat with your legs stretched out in front of you and shoulder width apart. Feet should be flexed, toes pointing to the ceiling. Keep your back and arms straight, with your arms by your sides and palms facing the mat.

2. Exhale. Draw in your abdominals, lower your chin to your chest and roll your upper spine down slowly as if peeling away from an imaginary wall. Glide your hands forward across the mat as you move, being mindful of keeping the shoulders down.

3. Inhale. Pause when you can't go any further and hold the position.

4. Exhale. Roll your spine back up that imaginary wall returning to the start position.

The Benefits

Strengthens the abdominals and back extensor muscles. Improves articulation of the spine and hamstring flexibility.

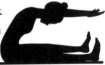

Tips and Technique Cues

- If you are unable to straighten your back with legs outstretched, modify the movement by bending your knees as much as needed to allow you to start with an upright spine.

- Keep your toes pointing up throughout and think of reaching forward with the heels.

- Keep your abdominals pulling inward as you flex your spine forward, visualizing a ball in your lap that you do not want to touch.

- Try to keep your pelvis still at the beginning of the exercise to emphasize the spinal flexion and articulation of the vertebrae – imagine someone with their arms around your waist gently stopping you tilting your pelvis forward.

- As you uncurl the spine, visualize stacking one vertebra directly on top of the other until you are fully upright once more.

- To increase the dynamics of the exercise when you are familiar with it, exhale to roll down and inhale to roll straight back up. Repeat 8–10 times.

Rolling Back

The Movement

Start position. Sit with your knees bent and feet close to your pelvis. Place your hands on your shins, draw your abdominals in and tilt your pelvis back slightly so you are able to lift both feet off the mat and balance. You are aiming to create a deep curve with the whole of your spine.

1. Draw your abdominals in further until you feel yourself start to tip backward.

2. Inhale. Maintain the shape of the body and roll back, stopping when you feel the weight on your shoulders and upper back.

3. Exhale to roll back up to the balance position without placing the feet down.

4. Repeat 8–10 times.

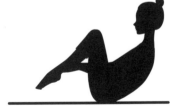

The Benefits

Builds abdominal strength and control. Increases skill in balance and muscle activation for whole body movement. Massages the spinal muscles.

Tips and Technique Cues

- If you have difficulty getting back to the start position, try holding your hands underneath your thighs for more support.

- Maintain the curved shape of the body throughout the exercise.

- To increase the challenge, bring your legs closer to your body and your head closer to your knees.

- To add variation place hands on the ankles and increase the lower back flexion while reducing the upper back flexion creating a more elongated curve.

Spine Twist

The Movement

1. Start position. Sit with your legs straight out in front of you, gently squeezing together. Flex your feet, with toes pointing toward the ceiling. Stretch your arms out to the sides, palms up, hands in line with the shoulders.

2. Exhale. Rotate the whole upper body gently to the right, then rotate a little further being mindful of keeping the movement gentle and controlled and your pelvis anchored onto the mat.

3. Inhale. Return to centre.

4. Exhale. Rotate upper body to the left gently, then rotate a little further.

5. Inhale. Return to centre.

6. Repeat 3–5 times on each side, 6–10 times in total.

The Benefits

Strengthens the abdominal oblique muscles. Teaches use of the core for rotation rather than momentum of arms and shoulders. Increases strength of the back extensors and creates mobility and flexibility in the spine.

Tips and Technique Cues

- If you have difficulty sitting with your legs straight, bend your knees.

- If you find it challenging keeping your legs together, place a ball or cushion between your knees.

- Keep your nose in line with the centre of your chest throughout so you are moving the torso as one unit.

- Initiate and control the movement from the waist rather than using your arms for momentum.

- Keep the legs and pelvis still throughout.

- Pull the abdominals in and up as you rotate to maintain an extended spine throughout.

Side Kick

The Movement

1. Start position. Lie on your side, propped up on one elbow with both your hands behind your head and fingers interlaced. Both legs should be straight, one on top of the other and slightly forward of your hips with the feet pointed. Raise the top leg to hip level.

2. Inhale. Swing your top leg forward and then slightly further forward, maintaining the height.

3. Exhale. Swing the leg back and then slightly further back. Repeat 6-10 times, change sides and do the same with the other leg.

The Benefits

Strengthens the hip flexors and extensors, the quadriceps and the ankle flexors. A great exercise to develop core stability as lying on your side makes it difficult to balance as there is less to balance on.

Also develops hip flexor and hamstring flexibility.

Tips and Technique Cues

- To modify, start with your bottom arm outstretched, head resting on your arm and other hand in front of your chest, palm down on the mat.

- Avoid both tilting the pelvis as the legs go forward and arching the back as the legs go back. When you feel any motion draw your abdominals in and up, and at the same time lift your waist away from the mat to initiate the stability required.

- To increase the challenge, stay propped up on your elbow but lift your ribcage completely off the mat and maintain this position throughout the exercise.

- Press your head back into your hands to maintain a neutral position of your cervical spine.

- For variation, you can flex the foot as the leg swings forward and point the toes as it goes back.

- You can also switch the breath pattern, exhaling forward and inhaling back.

Shoulder Bridge

The Movement

1. Start position. Lie on your back, knees bent, feet hip-width apart. Arms by your side, palms facing down.

2. Curl your pelvis up off the mat to the same place as you would for a pelvic curl. Now place your hands on the side of your waist, fingers pointing toward each other, elbows pressing into the floor to support the weight of your body. Lift your right foot off the mat, knee pointing to the ceiling and then unfold the leg so it is straight with toes pointed.

3. Exhale. Keep the leg straight and lower down toward the mat without letting your pelvis arch or your body change position.

4. Inhale. Lift the leg back up.
   Repeat five times.

5. Keep the body in the bridge position and bend the right leg at the knee and lower

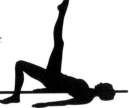

to the floor. Now unfold your left leg and repeat the sequence five times on this side.

6. Finish by rolling the spine back down onto the mat.

The Benefits

Increases hip flexor and hip extensor strength and flexibility – all the thigh and glute muscles. Increases core strength.

Tips and Technique Cues

- Focus on pulling the lower abdominals in and up to prevent the pelvis dropping.

- Be aware as you lower the leg of keeping your hips level and your abdominals engaged to maintain control.

- To increase the challenge remove your hands and place them palms down on the mat beside you for the whole exercise. This will also work your shoulder and spinal extensor muscles.

- For variation, try pointing the toes as you lower the leg and flexing the foot as you lift it back up – this will give you a dynamic hamstring stretch in the upward movement.

One Leg Stretch

The Movement

1. Start position. Lie on your back and pull your right knee into your chest, with your left hand placed just below the knee and your right hand holding the side of the shin just above the ankle. Lift your left leg to around 45 degrees, raise your head and chest up off the mat, eyeline forward toward your knee.

2. Inhale. Begin to bend the straight leg and at the same time begin to straighten the bent leg.

3. Exhale. Switch the legs so you now have a bent left leg and your right leg is outstretched. Your hands also need to switch so your right hand is below the knee and your left holding your shin.

4. Repeat the movement 6–10 times, making sure to exhale on each switch of the legs.

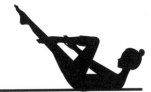

The Benefits

Targets the abdominals – rectus abdominis, external oblique and internal oblique. Also works the hip extensors and hip flexors. Builds skill in coordination of movement between legs, abdominals and arms.

Tips and Technique Cues

- Start by pulling your abdominal wall in so you set the intention and connection for the whole exercise.

- Keep your lower back and sacrum still on the mat throughout the switching of the legs.

- Think of constantly lifting your upper body up and forward while contracting your abdominals so you maintain the same height throughout the exercise rather than dropping back as the legs change position.

- Be aware of keeping your shoulders down throughout.

- To increase the challenge to the abdominals: when you bring your leg in, stop at the point where your knee is directly above your hip (rather than pulled in to your chest) and lower the opposite leg to just above the mat.

One Leg Kick

The Movement

1. Start position. Lie on your front with your upper body propped up on your forearms, elbows slightly forward of your shoulders. Fists lightly clenched and hands next to each other on the mat to form a triangle shape between your hands and two elbows. Legs are straight out behind you, slightly apart with feet pointed.

2. Draw your abdominal wall in and tilt your pelvis forward so you feel your hip bones tilt upward, away from the mat and an increased contraction in your abdominals. Lift the legs just off the floor, maintaining this abdominal connection.

3. Inhale. Bend the right knee with your heel coming toward your buttock.

4. Exhale. Switch the legs to bend the left leg with the heel coming toward your buttock.

5. Repeat this sequence 10 times making a total of 20 repetitions.

The Benefits

Strengthens hamstrings, the gluteus maximus, abdominals and the spinal extensor muscles. Increases abdominal control and builds the strength of the muscles that draw the shoulder blades down, scapula depressors.

Tips and Technique Cues

- If you feel discomfort in your back, take your elbows further out, or you can rest your head on your hands.

- It is very important to keep the abdominals pulling in and up, and the torso still throughout the entire exercise.

- Press the forearms down into the mat while simultaneously attempting to widen the space between your collar bones at the front and your shoulder blades at the back.

- Isolate the movement to your knees so the rest of your body is stable with a strong, extended spine.

- To increase the challenge to the spinal extensors and abdominals, bring your elbows in underneath your shoulders while maintaining the extension and the abdominal control.

I WAS 19 WHEN
I DISCOVERED PILATES,
AND I'M STILL DOING IT.
IT'S THE WORKOUT
MY BODY REALLY
RESPONDS TO.

Kate Hudson

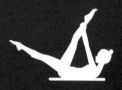

CHAPTER FOUR: INTERMEDIATE EXERCISES

This chapter takes you through the next
12 exercises of the Pilates repertoire. It is
recommended you learn the exercises one
by one and add them to the exercises from
the previous chapter. Moving through the
sequence from the beginning and if needed
starting with the modified options offered
will take your practice to the next level.

Double Leg Stretch

The Movement

1. Start position. Lying on your back, bring your legs to a tabletop position, nod your chin, lift your head, neck and chest up off the mat and place your hands on your knees.

2. Inhale. Reach both your arms down onto the sides of your legs in the direction of your feet while simultaneously extending both your legs straight out. Do this without lowering your torso and only extend out to an angle where you are able to keep your lower back pressing into the mat.

3. Exhale. Bend the legs and pull them back in to the tabletop position, replacing your hands just below the knees.

4. Repeat 6–10 times.

The Benefits

Increased abdominal strength and core stability. Increased strength and flexibility in the hip flexors.

Tips and Technique Cues

- Be sure to pull your abdominals in and up to maintain connection with the mat throughout the movement.

- To modify, try extending the legs at a higher angle, this will reduce the load on your hip flexors.

- To increase the abdominal challenge, reach your arms back overhead as far as you can without lowering your torso or moving your head. Exhale to circle the arms out to the side and back to the knees while simultaneously pulling your legs back in to the tabletop position.

- Keep your eyeline forward.

- Emphasize the exhale and drawing in of the legs to deepen the abdominal connection.

Saw

The Movement

1. Start position. Sit up on your mat with your back straight, legs out in front of you and a little wider than your shoulders. Flex your feet and hold your arms out to the side, in line with your shoulders. Palms facing down.

2. Inhale slowly. Keep your hips and pelvis still while rotating your upper body and arms toward the right, flex your spine forward, bringing your left arm across and toward the outside of your right foot.

3. Exhale slowly. Reaching your body forward three times in a saw-like motion. Straighten your spine and rotate back to the start position. Now repeat the sequence moving to the left.

4. Keep alternating sides and repeat 6–10 times in total.

The Benefits

Hamstring stretch. Abdominal oblique control and strength. Back extensor control.

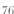

Tips and Technique Cues

- To modify the start position, bend your knees as much as you need so your spine is straight.

- This is a challenging movement both physically and for breath control so as another option you can increase the breaths to break the exercise down. Inhaling to rotate, exhaling to reach forward, inhaling to straighten the spine and exhaling to rotate back to the start position.

- Think of elongating your spine as you rotate to keep the back extensors engaged.

- When you reach forward, be very gentle, especially if you have flexibility challenges.

- You can vary the exercise by turning your palms forward to externally rotate and open up the shoulders.

- To reduce the emphasis on flexing the upper back and increase the hamstring stretch, you can keep your upper back in extension as you reach forward. This will deepen the flexion at your hips while increasing the stretch through the legs and lower back.

Rollover with Legs Spread

The Movement

1. Start position. Lie on your back with your arms down by your sides, palms down. Lift the legs and extend them so they are straight and at about 60 degrees to the mat (or higher if you are unable to hold them at this angle without your back arching).

2. Inhale. Bring the legs toward you to a 90-degree angle.

3. Exhale. Draw the abdominals in and bring your legs overhead, allowing your spine to curl up off the mat and your pelvis to lift and move toward the shoulders until it is floating above your chest. Your legs stay straight and parallel to the ceiling. This is the rollover position.

4. Inhale. Hold this position and lower your legs overhead toward the mat, touching it if your hamstring flexibility allows, then separate your legs to shoulder width apart.

5. Exhale. Slowly roll your spine, smoothly and with control, back onto the floor. Once your

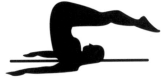

pelvis reconnects with the mat, lower the legs a little further down and then come back to your start position.

6. Repeat three times.

7. Now repeat the whole sequence reversing the leg position. Start with feet apart, roll over, lower legs, bring them together and roll back down. Repeat three times.

The Benefits

Spinal articulation, hamstring stretch, lower back stretch. Abdominal strength and control.

Tips and Technique Cues

* Avoid putting any pressure on your neck in the overhead position.

* Press your arms into the mat to help you stabilize, using your shoulders to assist.

* To modify the rollover phase, use your hands to support your pelvis in the rollover position.

* To vary the exercise, you can flex the feet in the overhead position to add further stretch to the hamstrings and the calf muscles.

Rocker with Open Legs

The Movement

1. Start position. Sit with your knees bent and apart, hands on the outside of your ankles and gently flex your lower back to enable you to float your feet up off the floor, gently pointed.

2. Extend your legs to straight, maintaining the hold of the ankles until your legs are in a V position. Your feet are shoulder width apart. Draw your abdominal wall in to initiate the backward tilt of your pelvis.

3. Inhale. Roll back onto your upper back while avoiding rolling as far as your neck. Exhale to roll forward and back up to the start position.

4. Repeat five times.

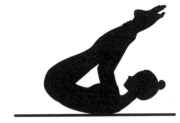

The Benefits

Strengthens all the abdominal muscles and hip flexors. Teaches control of the shoulders, arms and upper back muscles as well as the hip extensors.

Tips and Technique Cues

- To modify if flexibility is a challenge: bend your knees to a position you can hold without feeling tension in your hamstrings or lower back. You can also switch your hands to holding lower down the legs if needed.

- Think of the legs reaching away from you to help you come back up. Your arms will be holding them but the tension created between arms and hip extensors will help you roll back up.

- To increase the challenge, add a spinal extension at the end of each roll by holding onto the ankles, drawing your shoulders down and trying to lengthen and straighten your back. Be mindful of flexing from the lower back to initiate the next roll.

Corkscrew

The Movement

1. Start position. Lie on your back with your arms by your side, palms down. Perform a rollover so your legs are parallel to the floor, feet gently pointed.

2. Exhale. Move both legs to your right, twisting the body at your waist so your pelvis moves with your legs and your feet are pointing over your right shoulder.

3. Inhale. Lower the spine down while simultaneously drawing a circle with your feet, through centre and over to the left, lifting your spine back up to the rollover position to end the movement.

4. Exhale. Move both legs to your left, twisting the body at your waist so your pelvis moves with your legs and your feet are pointing over your left shoulder.

5. Inhale. Lower the spine down while simultaneously circling the legs down, through centre and over to the right, lifting

your spine back up to the rollover position to end the movement.

6. Repeat three times each side making six in total, alternating direction each time.

The Benefits

Builds strength through the abdominal obliques and rectus abdominis as well as working all the core muscles. Increases hip flexor strength as well as working hip extensors, hip adductors and all the major muscle groups of the legs.

Tips and Technique Cues

- To modify, perform the whole exercise lying on the mat allowing the legs, hips and pelvis to move in the corkscrew movement but maintaining contact between the pelvis and the mat. This is a great way to build control through the core and it is recommended to do it this way if you are unable to do the rollover.

- Move your pelvis and legs as one unit. Keep the legs pressing together.

- Keep your back pressing into the mat during the circle of the legs.

Side Bend

The Movement

1. Start position. Sit on your right hip with your knees bent, and the foot of your left leg in front of your right leg at the ankle. Your right arm is straight and propping you up, palm down on the mat. Rest your left arm on your left leg, close to the ankle with palm down.

2. Inhale. Lift the pelvis up, straightening your legs and lifting your top arm so fingers are pointing toward the ceiling creating a T shape.

3. Exhale. Lift higher while taking your top arm overhead to frame your face and simultaneously turning your head to look down toward the mat.

4. Inhale. Return the arm to point toward the ceiling and turn your head back to face front.

5. Exhale. Lower the body to the start position.

6. Repeat five times on each side.

The Benefits

Shoulder strength and stability, abdominal oblique strength and stretch.

Tips and Technique Cues

- Remember this is a side exercise so try not to rotate your body forward or back during any phase of the movement.

- Visualize making an arc with your body when you take the arm overhead, lifting the hips as far toward the ceiling as you can.

- To increase the challenge, once you lift up you can keep the legs straight. Inhale to lower the body until your bottom calf touches the mat while also turning your head to look toward your feet. Exhale to lift up, taking your arm overhead. Repeat five times each side. Please note this is very challenging to shoulder stability so only attempt this if you are confident in your ability to hold your weight safely on your shoulder.

Leg Pull Front

The Movement

1. Start position. In a plank position (we call this the Front Support in Pilates), with your knees and elbows straight, the crown of your head reaching out and slightly up, eyeline toward the front of your mat. Gently pull your abdominals in to stabilize the spine to prevent sinking into your lower back.

2. Inhale. Raise one leg toward the ceiling, gently pointing your toes while maintaining stillness in the spine.

3. Exhale to lower your leg back down and return to the plank position.

4. Inhale. Raise the opposite leg toward the ceiling, toes pointed.

5. Exhale to lower your leg down and return to the plank position. Repeat this sequence five times on each leg, 10 times in total.

The Benefits

Shoulder stability and strength. Glute, hamstring and abdominal strength.

Tips and Technique Cues

- To maintain stability through the shoulders, be sure to press the mat away with your hands in the plank position, this will help activate the shoulder stabilizer muscles.

- Visualize the leg reaching away as you lift it, being mindful of keeping your knee straight at all times.

- The pelvis stays neutral so lifting the leg must be done with control, to ensure you do not rotate your pelvis in the direction of the leg that is lifting; both hip bones should stay facing the mat.

- If painful to the wrists you can modify the exercise by doing the plank position on your forearms.

Swimming

The Movement

1. Start position. Lie on your front with your arms straight out overhead and your legs also straight.

2. Raise both your legs together just off the floor while simultaneously raising your arms, head and chest off the floor. Keep your knees and elbows straight, and point your toes.

3. Maintaining the position of your spine, raise the right arm and left leg a little higher.

4. Switch to raising the left arm and right leg a little higher, creating a swimming motion.

5. Continue to switch the movements from side to side in a swift yet controlled motion for ten breaths.

The Benefits

This is an excellent exercise for working the whole back of the body, calf muscles, hamstrings, glutes, spinal extensors and rotators and shoulders. All these actions are used when walking and running and in many other movements so it is invaluable for developing torso rotational stability.

Tips and Technique Cues

- Be mindful of keeping your abdominal connection throughout by constantly pulling in and up on your lower abdominals so as not to overarch your back.

- Keep elbows and knees straight at all times.

- Think of the legs being light, reaching out and just fluttering at speed as if swimming in water.

- Keep the legs from touching the floor at any point in the exercise.

- To increase the challenge, add the breath pattern of the Hundred exercise (see page 52). Inhale for 5 counts, then exhale for 5 counts until you have completed 10 breath cycles.

Side Kick Kneeling

The Movement

1. Start position. This is a more advanced version of the Side Kick from the beginners' exercise chapter (see page 64). Start by kneeling up, placing your left leg out to the side on the mat, foot pointed. Flex your torso sideways in the opposite direction, place your right hand on the mat, palm down to support you and your left hand behind your head. Raise your left leg up until it is in line with your hip.

2. Inhale. Bring the leg forward keeping the foot in line with your hip.

3. Exhale to bring the leg back again keeping that alignment.

4. Repeat five times, then change to the other side and repeat the sequence.

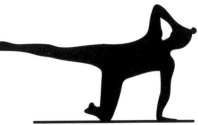

The Benefits

Strengthens the spinal lateral flexors and stabilizers, all the abdominal muscles and the outer thigh muscles including the glutes. Increases strength in the shoulders.

Tips and Technique Cues

- Press your supporting hand into the mat to help stabilize the shoulder.

- Think of lifting upward continually to encourage the use of the core to keep the torso stable so it neither arches or flexes while the leg moves forward and back.

- To modify, if you find it difficult to hold your leg at hip height, lower the leg to a level you can hold and maintain control to perform the movement.

- To increase the challenge, bring the swinging leg higher to increase the work of the outer hip muscles.

- For variation, you can add a change of foot position; flex the foot as the leg swings forward and point it as it goes back. You can also add a double leg pulse, pulsing forward for two counts and back for two counts while continuing to stay stable in your back.

Teaser

The Movement

1. Start position. Lie on your back and lift your legs into tabletop position, then straighten them to an angle of 60 degrees. Keep your legs pressing together and your toes gently pointed. Raise your arms, palms down, to the same angle so arms and legs are parallel. Raise your head and chest until shoulder blades are off the floor.

2. Inhale. Draw your abdominals in and curl your spine up off the mat until you are balancing on your buttocks. Move your arms forward with you to maintain their position parallel to the legs. Your legs should not move at all.

3. Exhale. Curl the spine back down to the start position.

4. Repeat five times.

The Benefits

Increases abdominal and hip flexor strength. Builds endurance and increases spinal articulation while also improving balance.

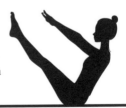

Tips and Technique Cues

- This is a very challenging exercise, so if you feel any strain in your back it is recommended you modify the movement by keeping your legs bent and draw them in a little closer to your body. You can also hold on to the back of your legs to reduce the intensity further.

- Concentrate on pulling your abdominals in, to maintain stability as well as keeping a smooth movement of the spine as you curl up and down.

- Imagine someone is holding your ankles so your legs remain completely still throughout the movement.

- Avoid lifting your shoulders in your quest to reach forward, keep pressing them down.

- Move the arms and legs in parallel throughout the movement.

- To increase the challenge, raise your arms at the end of each movement to add spinal extension to the movement. Lower your arms as you curl down and take them overhead, then bring them forward, curl up and lift them overhead.

Leg Pull

The Movement

1. Start position. Sit on your mat with your legs outstretched in front of you and gently squeezing together, feet pointed. Keeping your arms straight, place your hands on the mat behind you, fingers pointing out to the side. Lengthen and straighten your spine to engage both abdominals and back muscles.

2. Lift your pelvis up off the mat creating a straight line through the front of your body - ankles, knees, hips and shoulders in a diagonal line. This is a reverse plank.

3. Inhale. Raise the right leg up toward the ceiling.

4. Exhale. Lower the leg back onto the mat.

5. Inhale. Raise the left leg up toward the ceiling.

6. Exhale. Lower the leg back down to the mat.

7. Repeat five times on each leg.

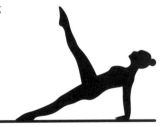

The Benefits

A powerful exercise that builds strength in the muscles on the back of the body through having to stabilize and hold the position. Builds strength and flexibility in the hip flexors and extensors during the leg lift and lower.

Tips and Technique Cues

- Press your arms down to emphasize shoulder stability.

- Press your toes toward the floor as you lift and maintain the sense of length through the leg. Be mindful of keeping your legs straight but avoid them being over straightened, so as not to strain your knee joint.

- If you feel any discomfort in the back of your knee, it is recommended you bend the knee of your supporting leg while lifting and lowering the other leg.

- To modify, start building strength by lifting into the reverse plank position without the leg lift. Once you feel strong enough to hold the position, add the leg lift.

- To increase the challenge, perform 5 repetitions on the right leg, then 5 on the left.

Swan Dive

The Movement

1. Start position. Lie on your front, propped up on your forearms as you did for One Leg Kick (see page 70). Engage your abdominals, pulling inward and upward to avoid sinking into your lower back. Keep your legs straight and hip-width apart, feet pointed.

2. Inhale. Straighten your arms, lifting your chest higher off the mat. At the same time raise your legs, keeping the knees straight so your body is in an arc position. Hold this shape.

3. Exhale. Rock the body forward, gently bending the elbows.

4. Inhale. Rock the body back, straightening the elbows.

5. Repeat the sequence five times. When you have mastered this preparation movement successfully, take your arms out to the side on the first inhale and leave them there throughout

the five repetitions of the movement, so you are rocking forward and back without your arms for assistance.

6. Finish by placing the hands on the mat and bringing the chest back down.

The Benefits

Increases muscle tone and endurance through the back of the body, in particular the spinal extensors and the hip extensors.

Tips and Technique Cues

- This is a high-risk exercise to the back so it is advised to start with the modified version below or the preparation movement above, and only attempt the full movement when you are confident in the strength of your back and the ability to hold the torso in extension.

- To increase the challenge further you can reach your arms overhead instead of out to the side, maintaining this position throughout the five repetitions.

I DO AN HOUR
OF PILATES A DAY.
IT IS FANTASTIC AND
FITNESS-WISE I AM
THE BEST I HAVE BEEN
FOR A LONG TIME.

David Beckham

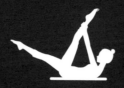

CHAPTER FIVE:
ADVANCED EXERCISES

It is strongly advised before attempting any of the exercises in this chapter that you are able to perform all of the exercises from the previous two chapters competently and with confidence in your ability to control your body. The advanced exercises require a very high level of athletic ability, control and flexibility. Where there is a modified option, it is recommended you start with that and progress from there.

Neck Pull

The Movement

1. Start position. Lie on your back in a neutral position with your legs straight, feet flexed and hands behind your head, fingers interlaced.

2. Inhale. Draw your lower abdominals inward to engage the core and gently nod your chin to your chest. Lift your head and chest up, so your shoulder blades are off the mat.

3. Exhale. Continue lifting, the same as you would do for a Roll Up, until your spine is curled forward and your chest is over your legs in a deep stretch position.

4. Inhale. Begin to roll back in a rounded C position.

5. Exhale. Complete the roll back until you are back to the start position on the mat. Repeat 10 times.

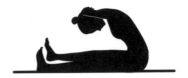

The Benefits

Increases the challenge to the abdominals having to keep the hands behind the head. Improves spinal articulation of the back, as more attention is needed to execute the exercise without the help of the arms. Improves flexibility on both the hamstrings and the back extensors.

Tips and Technique Cues

- To modify, you can begin the exercise by reaching your arms forward at the point you find it difficult to curl up, replacing the hands behind the head as soon as you are comfortably up.

- To increase the challenge, instead of rolling back in a C curve, unroll the spine to an upright position and keeping the back straight, hinge back from the hips maintaining a straight back for as long as you are able to hold it. Then draw in deeper on the abdominals to flex your lower back and curl back down to the mat.

- You can also add variation by flexing the feet as an alternative position.

Hip Twist

The Movement

1. Start position. Sit on the mat with your arms placed behind you to a distance where you feel your weight is back over your pelvis with your spine remaining straight. Fingers are pointing away from your body, chest open. Bend your knees and, keeping them together, lift and extend the legs straight out to create a V position.

2. Exhale. Rotate your pelvis to the right, moving both legs at the same time in a circular motion to the right, down and across to centre.

3. Inhale. Continue this small circular movement by bringing your legs up to the left and rotating the pelvis to the left. And then returning the legs to centre and the pelvis back to the start position.

4. Exhale. Shift the legs and pelvis to the left, circling the legs down and across to centre.

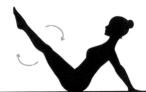

5. Inhale. Continue the circle bringing the legs and pelvis to the right and back to the start position.

6. Repeat three times each side making a total of six movements.

The Benefits

Builds strength and competency in rotation and stabilization. In particular utilizing the hip flexors, spinal flexors and rotators.

Tips and Technique Cues

- Press downward into the mat to encourage scapular stabilization and a strong base of support through the upper body.

- Keep the leg circles small enough to be able to control the stability in your back, preventing the back from arching and the pelvis from tilting.

- To modify, bend the knees as much as needed if you feel any strain in your lower back or hamstrings.

- To add variation, switch your breathing: beginning with an inhale to shift your legs, followed by an exhale to perform the circle.

Jack Knife

The Movement

1. Start position. Lie on your back, arms by your side, palms down. Lift your legs so they are straight and at a 60-degree angle to the mat (or higher if you feel your back arching.) Point your toes.

2. Inhale. Bring your legs to 90 degrees. Roll over, lifting your pelvis and lower back off the mat, taking your legs overhead to a diagonal line above your face and then extending the back further into a vertical line, toes pointing toward the ceiling.

3. Exhale. Slowly roll your torso down as smoothly as possible. Once your pelvis touches the mat, return your legs to the start position.

4. Repeat five times.

The Benefits

Increases the challenge to spinal extension as it includes deeper spinal articulation by moving through flexion into extension as the legs lift up. Increases flexibility in the hamstrings and lower back muscles. Increases muscle strength in the hip extensors.

Tips and Technique Cues

- When taking your legs overhead, do not allow them to drop, keep them lifted, maintaining a space between them and your face before lifting up to the ceiling.

- As you lift your legs to the vertical position, simultaneously press your arms down into the mat to help encourage the lift and extension of your spine as well as supporting your body weight on your shoulders.

- To modify, you can place your hands on the back of your pelvis, creating a shoulder stand position and bring the legs as far over as your hamstrings will allow. This also reduces the weight-bearing aspect on your neck.

- To add a further challenge, lower the legs to touch the floor at the end of the rollover before lifting to the vertical line.

Control Balance

The Movement

1. Start position. Do a Rollover with Legs Spread (see page 78). Hold the position with your legs overhead and feet touching the ground. Circle your arms around and overhead to take hold of the sides of the feet.

2. Exhale. Move your hands so one is holding your left ankle and the other is holding your left calf, while simultaneously raising your right leg toward the ceiling until it is vertical.

3. Inhale. Let go of your left leg and switch the leg and hand positions, so you are now holding your right leg with your left leg extended toward the ceiling.

4. Repeat three times on each leg, alternating sides to make six times in total.

5. To finish, bring both feet down toward your head before rolling the spine back on to the mat.

The Benefits

An extremely challenging movement, this exercise teaches control of the core to maintain balance and control in inversion. It builds strength in both spinal flexors and extensors, as well as increasing hip extensor strength and flexibility.

Tips and Technique Cues

- Keep the weight of your body on the shoulders, as this exercise poses a high risk to the neck.

- Keep a sense of length in the curved position of your spine so you do not let your body weight collapse onto your neck. Visualize your tailbone reaching up to the ceiling.

- Reach your leg away slowly, so as to maintain control of the body in hip extension – as your torso will want to roll back toward the mat.

- To increase the challenge, perform two gentle pulses of your leg when it is extended to the ceiling, hold this position for two breaths, then inhale to switch legs and repeat.

Double Kick

The Movement

1. Start position. Lie on your front with your legs together, hands behind your back, elbows bent and one hand holding the other. Rest your hands on your sacrum and allow your elbows to drop toward the floor. Turn your head to one side and rest your cheek on the mat.

2. Tense the muscles of the back of the legs and bottom and lift your legs just off the floor, keeping your knees straight and feet pointed.

3. Exhale. Bend both knees and bring your heels swiftly toward your bottom.

4. Inhale. Raise your chest off the mat, straightening your elbows, lifting your arms and bringing your head in line with the rest of your spine. Simultaneously straighten your legs, reaching them out and up toward the ceiling.

5. Return to the start position, turning your head to rest on the other cheek.

6. Repeat six times, alternating your head position at the end of each movement.

The Benefits

Increases back strength and flexibility. Increases glute and hamstring strength. Gives a dynamic stretch to the shoulder flexors. Great for anyone who works at a desk.

Tips and Technique Cues

- Keep the abdominals pulling in and up throughout the exercise to reduce arching in your lower back.

- Visualize your spine lifting to form a gentle arc from the base of your skull to the tips of your toes.

- Keep your legs pressed together throughout.

- Use your glute muscles to lift your legs in a straight position at the start of the exercise.

- To modify, if you feel any discomfort in your back, start with your legs resting on the mat, raise them to kick and then lower them back to the mat.

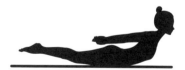

Scissors

The Movement

1. Start position. Lie on your back and perform a rollover (see page 78). Bend your knees and place your hands on the back of your pelvis, fingers pointing away from your head. Gently lower the weight of your pelvis into your hands, creating a slight arch of your back. Extend your legs vertically, keeping them straight and reaching toward the ceiling.

2. Inhale to lower one leg toward your face and the other leg away in the opposite direction to form a scissor position.

3. Exhale. Switch legs so they go in opposite directions, creating a scissor position once again.

4. Repeat 10 times in total.

The Benefits

Deepens the flexibility of both the hip flexors and extensors. Stretching of the hip flexors is particularly

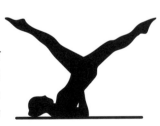

helpful for those who spend much of the day seated. Increases core strength and spinal stability.

Tips and Technique Cues

- While your legs are moving, keep the rest of your body completely still.

- Pull in and up on the front of your lower abdominals to encourage core connection and stabilization of the pelvis.

- Press your elbows down into the mat to encourage use of the shoulder extensors, and gently draw your shoulder blades toward each other to prevent the shoulders from rounding forward.

- To modify, place your hands lower on your back and decrease the arch to neutral if needed, to release any instability or discomfort in your back.

- To increase the challenge, add a double pulse of both legs in the scissor position, exhaling on the pulses and then inhaling to switch the legs over. With each exhale, try to reach your legs further from the centre to increase the stretch, while keeping your pelvis still and stable.

Bicycle

The Movement

1. Start position. Begin in the same way as the Scissors (see page 110) with your legs in the scissor position. Right leg overhead and left leg reaching the opposite way.

2. Inhale. Bend your left leg, bringing your toes toward the mat.

3. Exhale. Bring that same leg in toward your chest with your knee bent while the right leg stays straight and lowers toward the mat, finishing with the bent leg unfolding so you are back in the scissor position.

4. Inhale. Bend your right leg.

5. Exhale. Bring that knee in while the left leg stays straight and lowers toward the mat, finishing with the top leg unfolding to straight so you are back in the scissor position once again.

6. Repeat 10 times in total, then reverse the direction of the movement for 10 repetitions.

The Benefits

As with the Scissors, this deepens the flexibility of both the hip flexors and hip extensors but with increased challenge to stability of the core and coordination of the mind and body to create a smooth sequence of movement.

Tips and Technique Cues

- Think of riding a bike slowly uphill so you create a controlled and steady movement.

- Pull in and up on the front of your lower abdominals to encourage core connection and stability of the pelvis.

- Press your elbows down into the mat to encourage your shoulders to stabilize your upper body.

- To modify, place your hands lower on your back and decrease the arch to neutral if needed, to release any instability or discomfort in your back.

- To increase the challenge, perform the exercise with an increased arch of the back, with the intention of being able to touch the toes of your bottom leg onto the mat.

Rocking

The Movement

1. Start position. Lie on your front, knees close together and bent. Reach your hands behind you, taking hold of your ankles.

2. Lift your head and chest away from the mat and at the same time reach your feet away and up toward the ceiling, so your knees also lift away from the mat.

3. Inhale. Hold this position and rock your body forward, visualizing your head, body and thighs as forming the same shape as the base of a rocking chair.

4. Exhale. Rock your body back, still holding the position of the body.

5. Repeat 10 times.

The Benefits

Increases flexibility in the shoulder, hip and spinal extensors. Increases back extensor strength, endurance and core stability. Another great

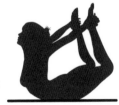

exercise to counteract the daily posture of rounded shoulders and flexed spine associated with sitting at a desk for long hours.

Tips and Technique Cues

- Initiate the rocking motion by lifting your knees a little higher and use the shoulder extensors to pull your feet up and forward. To rock back, place the emphasis on extending your spine and lifting the front of your body up which will switch the gravitational pull and bring your back to the start position.

- To modify, start with your chest down, knees bent and close together, holding onto each foot with one hand. Inhale to raise your head and chest away from the mat while simultaneously reaching your toes toward the ceiling. Only go as far as to feel a good stretch in the front of your thighs and no discomfort in your lower back. Exhale to lower back to the mat.

- At all times keep your abdominals engaged by pulling in and up so as to control the tilt of your pelvis to a range which is comfortable.

Boomerang

The Movement

1. Start position. Sit on your mat with your legs out in front of you, one foot crossed over the other at ankle level. Put your hands by your sides, palms down with fingers pointing forward. Arms and back are straight.

2. Exhale. Roll your body back onto the mat allowing your legs to lift into the rollover position. Switch legs so your feet are crossed the other way.

3. Inhale. Roll forward and up into a Teaser position (see page 92), taking your arms behind you with palms facing up.

4. Exhale. Lower your legs to the mat, bring your head down toward your knees while your arms reach further up and back.

5. Inhale. Hold the position of your body as the arms circle around to the front.

6. Exhale. Roll your spine back and go straight into step 2.

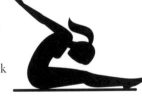

7. Repeat the sequence six times, switching legs each time.

8. To finish, unroll your spine to the start position.

The Benefits

This movement is a fusion of everything you have learnt previously with the Roll Up, the Rollover with Legs Spread, the Teaser and the Spine Stretch. It teaches endurance, control, coordination and core stability to create a sophisticated movement.

Tips and Technique Cues

- If your hamstrings are too tight to have your legs straight, you can bend your knees a little as you roll up to the V position. This will limit any strain on the lower back.

- To increase the challenge, come into a fully extended spine in the V position and bring your arms overhead for the Teaser position (step 3). Hold your legs still as you take your arms behind you, interlace your fingers and reach your arms out for a shoulder stretch. Then continue with step 4.

Seal

The Movement

1. Start position. Sit with your knees bent and apart, feet just touching each other at the toes.

2. Place your hands through the centre of your legs, under them and onto the outside of each ankle. Gently flex your lower back to create a C curve of your spine and float your feet up, holding on to them while balancing on your sit bones. Maintain this shape.

3. Inhale. Roll back onto your upper back.

4. Exhale. Roll up, bringing your body to the start position and clap your feet together twice.

5. Repeat 10 times.

The Benefits

Like Rolling Back (see page 60), this exercise requires control of the abdominals and spinal muscles to maintain the C curve of your spine, so the roll is both smooth and

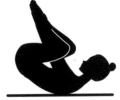

steady. Adding the clap of your feet at the end of each movement challenges this control further, as well as your ability to keep the movement going using the abdominals to initiate each roll back.

Tips and Technique Cues

- Use your abdominal muscles to create the tilt back and the C curve from your head to your tailbone.

- Pull your abdominals in deeper as you roll back and try to keep the shape of your body the same throughout the exercise.

- To modify, hold your legs on the outside under your knees or the insides of your feet, but keep them apart as you familiarize yourself with the movement. This also allows for any inflexibility you may feel in your legs or hips.

- To increase the challenge, clap three times at the beginning of the exercise and also when balanced on your shoulders.

Crab

The Movement

1. Start position. Sit on your mat with your knees bent,
   one ankle crossed over the other and holding onto your
   feet with the opposite hand. Each hand cradles the foot
   from the inside. Gently draw your abdominals in and
   tilt your pelvis back, lifting your feet off the floor to
   balance on your sit bones.

2. Inhale. Roll back holding this shape, swiftly switch the
   legs so the ankles are crossed the opposite way.

3. Exhale. Roll back up to the start position.

4. Repeat six times.

The Benefits

Strengthens the abdominal muscles, improves
coordination in many muscles thanks to the challenge of
maintaining your position as your legs switch. In the full
exercise the challenge of rolling forward over the knees
stretches the spinal extensors and requires a deeper level
of abdominal control so as not to land on your head.

Tips and Technique Cues

- Keep your thighs close to your chest and knees toward the inside of your shoulders.

- The original version of this exercise is high risk to anyone with neck, spine or knee issues. If you're ready for the challenge, roll back as before, switch the legs and then roll forward over the legs, drawing the abdominals in and up, hips to the ceiling and gently resting the top of the head on the floor. Tuck the chin slightly to elongate the back of the neck while continuing to lift up with the abdominals to minimize the weight on the neck bones.

- If doing the original version, make sure your head is placed down gently with control and a sense of resistance so as not to put unnecessary pressure on your neck bones.

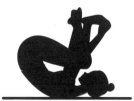

Push-Up

The Movement

1. Start position. Stand with your feet hip-width apart and roll your body down, bringing your hands onto the mat. Walk your hands forward until you are in the Front Support position (see page 86).

2. Inhale. Bend your elbows, keeping them close to the side of your body and lower your chest toward the mat.

3. Exhale. Straighten your elbows and return to Front Support. Do two more push-ups, lift your hips to the ceiling and walk your hands back to your feet. Unroll your spine back up to standing.

4. Repeat the sequence five times.

The Benefits

A full body-strengthening exercise that focuses on abdominals, shoulder stability and strength, spinal flexion and extension, hip extension and flexion, as well as dynamic stretch of the hamstring muscles.

Tips and Technique Cues

When moving into Front Support, be careful not to let your pelvis drop down or lift up too much. This will keep your lower back strong and stable.

- Imagine pressing the mat away with your hands to stabilize your shoulders.

- Keep your elbows close to your sides and pointing back as you lower your chest toward the mat.

- To modify, if hamstring flexibility prevents your hands reaching the floor, bend your knees as much as needed to be able to place your palms on the mat.

- If you are unable to do the full push-up without losing control of your shoulders or core form, reduce the bend of the elbows to a range you can control. Or, simply practise holding the position before coming back up.

Conclusion

This book has covered the background, guiding principles and exercises to give you all you need to start practising confidently at home. Now you have a greater understanding of how the body works and how using your mind can also bring a deeper sense of well-being to your daily movement.

Remember with Pilates, less is more! You do not have to do all the exercises in this book, there is no rush to reach the end, nor do you even need to advance to the more difficult movements. This is your guide; use it to help you progress to where feels right for you, and always listen to your body.

Keep in mind the principles of breath, concentration, centre, control, precision and flow as you move through each movement. And most of all, enjoy the sense of fulfilment you get by practising on a regular basis. Remember you are a unique being and your Pilates experience is unique to you. What unites you with Pilates fans all over the world is the sheer joy of moving your body for a fitter, healthier, happier you. Enjoy your practice, be mindful and never stop moving!

Index

THE LITTLE BOOK OF BREATHWORK

Jo Peters

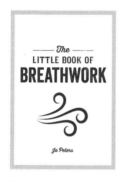

Paperback
ISBN: 978-1-80007-708-9

Learn how to use the power of your breath to gain clarity, peace and better health with this beginner's guide to the ancient practice of breathwork. *The Little Book of Breathwork* contains an overview of the history of breathwork and step-by-step instructions for carrying out different techniques safely in your own home.

Have you enjoyed this book? If so, find us
on Facebook at **Summersdale Publishers**,
on Twitter at **@Summersdale** and on Instagram
at **@summersdalebooks** and get in touch.
We'd love to hear from you!

www.summersdale.com

Image Credits

pp.3, 9, 27, 51, 73, 92, 99, 128, 40, 52, 54, 55, 56, 58, 60, 64, 68,
70, 76, 80, 82, 84, 86, 88, 94, 100, 108, 118, 120, 122 © a-yun/
Shutterstock.com; p.33 © Arcady/Shutterstock.com; pp.42, 74,
78 © Robert Davies/Shutterstock.com; p.44 © crack studio/
Shutterstock.com; pp.46, 48 © solar22/Shutterstock.com; pp.66, 106
© Elizabeta Lexa/Shutterstock.com; p.90 © Bojanovic/Shutterstock.
com; p.102 © Baleika Tamara/Shutterstock.com; p.104 © Bipsun/
Shutterstock.com; p.114 © Christos Georghiou/Shutterstock.com;
p.116 © graphixmania/Shutterstock.com